HEALING YOURSELF

A 32-DAY PROGRAM

Betty Lynn Tims

ISBN: 9781688312685

DEDICATION

This book is dedicated to the neurologist who directed me to my
meditation practice.

CONTENTS

ACKNOWLEDGMENTS

I would like to acknowledge all the great spiritual teachers
who have been in my life from youth group leaders,
Catholic priests, and Buddhist teachers and authors, as well
as countless meditation and yoga teachers.
Your work matters. Thank you.

CHAPTER ONE

Your faith in God may have been recently disrupted by illness or disease. Perhaps you abandoned hope a long time ago. For if God is good and created all things then why did he create illness? You are on the journey to understand why. This book is intended as a guide to coping with and understanding illness through contemplation, meditation, journaling, prayer and carefully crafted writing exercises.

Imagine a life without disease and illness. You are also imagining a life without love, hope, the sun, the moon, and the stars. Because all of these are God's creations, we must accept them wholeheartedly. It is when we react to disease and illness with fear, hatred, and anger that it becomes our poison. When we react to unfortunate circumstances such as illness with love, patience, and contentment the disease itself becomes our own medicine.

Illness can also become our teacher. It teaches us humility. It teaches us to be grateful for the small things. It teaches us to see the love in our caretaker's eyes. It teaches us to have patience and tolerance. And it opens our eyes to the suffering of others. Disease may be your greatest teacher and the fruits of these lessons will give you the grace you need to live the life God intended for you on earth.

When I was first diagnosed with my illness, I had lost all faith in God. I failed to see all the blessings around me: the patience in my doctor's eyes, the love with which my mother held my hand, and the time with which I was blessed. I only felt despair and anger with God. "How could you do this to me?!?! I was PERFECT! You ruined everything!" I felt that way for years and had a huge pity party. I could rejoice in nothing and was so numb with grief that I don't think I shed a single tear over my diagnosis.

That was seven years ago. Now today most people I know don't even know that I live with an illness. I no longer see myself as the patient, but a student-a student of life. It has taught me that I can still enjoy life. I have moved away from fear.

Fear-based thought is the biggest enemy. If you have a fear-based thought, say a quick prayer, "May I move out of fear and into faith." Fear can take us to places that we would never want to go. As long as we go there in our minds, we live that reality. Our mind becomes polluted and we feel trapped. There is no way out of this trap-except that the trap is an illusion we have built ourselves. This program is like a sledgehammer for the traps in our mind.

We must not live in fear. It doesn't matter what our circumstances are. This was not God's intention for us.

Suffering, fear, desire for better circumstances all may have created a mental trap of which we feel that we may never come free of. Maybe we are not even aware that we are living in this negative mental formation. However, with contemplation, prayer, written exercises and journaling we can do a series of things:

- We can recognize and raise awareness of the trap.
- We can see how it is made by recurring thoughts and fears.
- We can deconstruct the trap by formally interrupting the thought patterns or mental formations through meditation, contemplation, journaling, written exercises and prayer.

Think of a tree whose main branch gets cut off. What happens? The other branches get stronger and bigger. That is what illness and disease can do. You can turn them into your poison or your medicine. Disease is a great teacher for the willing student. This program begins your path to freedom. Not from disease but from the emotional suffering associated with disease.

Emotional suffering can be a trauma in and of itself. The disease may affect the body or the mind, but emotional suffering wreaks havoc on your spiritual equanimity. You may not be able to change your physical conditions. However, you can change the way you relate to them. It is your choice. In any given situation, in any given circumstance, you may find joy or you may find sorrow. The situation itself is negligible. However, your reaction is not. This is true in life. This is also true with illness and disease. Choose life, chose joy. Live the way that is pleasing to God.

This book will help you practice 7 key dimensions of our true reality: love, abundance, gratefulness, forgiveness, compassion, self-love, happiness, and God's divine plan. All of these are God's will for us. All of these should be part of a daily practice.

CHAPTER TWO

This is a 32-day program. Each day you should contemplate the meditation, pray earnestly, reflect in your journal, and complete the written exercises. This should take 20-30 minutes to complete. Do it in the morning, afternoon, or evening or whatever time suits you best. Throughout the day, when facing difficulty, pain, boredom, or any other challenge, remind yourself of the mantra. A mantra is something that you say to yourself over and over again in order to engrain it into your spiritual fabric and being. After 8 days is over repeat this cycle three more times. In about a month you will have grown significantly in a spiritual sense.

When you contemplate one of the meditations, take at least 10 minutes to do the following: memorize it, repeat it to yourself, and interpret it (put it in your own words and ask yourself, "What does this mean to me?") Thoughts will naturally arise during this process. It is important that you write them down during the reflection. Your understanding of certain ideas and concepts will deepen through the program. Your reflections in your journal will show your progress in coming to realizations and affirmations.

During traditional meditation you have an object to focus on such as the breath. However, during the meditations that follow, the written words will be your object of meditation. Therefore, you will steady your attention and focus your mind on the words of the meditation. These will resonate within your heart, mind, and soul. As you go throughout your day and week these will continue to affect your disposition as a stone that has sunk beneath the water continues to ripple the surface. Each meditation is like another stone.

The ripple effects of a 32-day program can be profoundly life-changing. These meditations will grant you the ability to develop a refined wisdom within your heart and mind that may then answer the question, "Why did God create illness and disease?" You will come to an understanding of your situation that was previously impossible. As Martin Luther King said, "Darkness cannot drive out darkness; only light can do that. Hate cannot drive out hate; only love can do that." Once you invite the love into your life once more the burden of illness will be slowly lifted. Like a veil is being lifted from your eyes you will see clearly a bright new day and experience freedom from the slavery of suffering. Suffering is only a state of mind. Once you decide to choose happiness instead of suffering despite your illness or disease you will experience freedom. Happiness naturally arises from stillness. The more you invest in your spiritual health the greater your spiritual wealth will be.

During contemplation of the meditation, painful or disturbing thoughts may arise. As you work through these difficult parts of your mind's current state, it is better to acknowledge them, see them for what they are (fears) and let them dissolve away as you work your way back to the meditation. Of course, if you are experiencing suicidal thoughts you should seek immediate professional help. However, if the thought or feeling is less serious it is best to stay present with it, acknowledge it and shift your focus back to the meditation. You might find that there are feelings, ideas, fears, or even terrors that exist beneath the surface of your consciousness that you were unaware of. It is important to recognize these thoughts as this will raise awareness of your current mental formations and thought patterns.

In Tibet, monks and nuns offer up prayers of gratitude for suffering. They want to make sure that they have enough suffering to be able to cultivate wisdom and compassion (Kornfield, Guided Meditations CD, gratitude intro) The aim of spiritual life according to Jack Kornfield is to awaken a joyful freedom, a benevolent and compassionate heart in the midst of all things. In the West we have achieved a level of material wealth that is astounding. People want for nothing yet find themselves feeling empty, lost, anxiety-ridden and have no sense of self. They have forgotten that they are a child of God. Disease, if treated rightly, can be

God's way of calling you back into his presence. My meditation teacher says, "Prayer is when you speak and God listens. Meditation is when God speaks and you listen."

It is important to sit quietly with yourself. With all your suffering, trauma, pain, and grief…sit. You may even find at the end of this program that you count your illness as a blessing. I know I do. After all, would you normally have taken the time to cultivate a daily practice in which you infuse your life with love, happiness, compassion, forgiveness, gratefulness, abundance, and God's divine plan for you? Or would you be going about your daily routine pursuing aimless activities with reckless abandon?

This program is a choice you chose. You chose wisdom over futility. You chose love over hate. You chose abundance over infertile visions of yourself. You chose life, joy, and light. Take my word for it: Disease can bring all these blessings to your heart's door. Just be kind to yourself and invite them in. Make an altar for them in your heart's center. Let your heart open and bloom like a rose in a beautiful garden. Let your soul sing.

CHAPTER THREE

Eight Meditations for 32 Days

1. <u>Self-identification</u>

"I am not an illness. I am a person living with an illness. Inside me is my true being, perfect and free from illness. I exist above the realm of illness."

Recommended Prayer Time: 5 minutes

Journal: Reflection

Exercise: List 10 things you like about yourself.

Mantra for the day: I am healthy.

2. <u>Gratefulness</u>

"Instead of seeing my illness as a burden, I will be grateful for all that it has brought me. It has brought me many people to support me. It has brought me humility. I can understand other's suffering better. It has brought me back to God."

Recommended Prayer Time: 5 minutes

Journal: Reflection

Exercise: List ten things you are grateful for

Mantra for the day: I am grateful.

3. <u>Love</u>

"I love my (insert affected body part, or simply "body"). God's light is inside my (insert affected body part, or simply "body"). I can see light healing my (insert affected body part, or simply "body"). My (insert affected body part, or simply "body") is free from disease.

Recommended Prayer Time: 5 minutes

Journal: Reflection

Exercise: List ten things you love about your body

Mantra for the day: My body is full of light.

4. <u>**Abundance**</u>

"I am healthy in many ways. God has blessed my body so that it may function in the way it does now. I can breathe. Therefore, I experience God's creation. I am alive and blessed with abundance."

Recommended Prayer Time: 5 minutes

Journal: Reflection

Exercise: List ten ways in which you are abundantly healthy.

Mantra for the day: I am blessed with abundance.

5. <u>**Forgiveness**</u>

"I forgive myself for having (illness). It is not my fault. I forgive God for making this part of my life. I understand that this is part of my journey to wisdom and freedom."

Recommended Prayer Time: 10 minutes

Journal: Reflection

Exercise: List ten good things that have happened since your diagnosis.

Mantra for the day: Forgiveness leads to freedom.

6. __Happiness__

"There are many ways to be happy. There can be suffering in life and I can still be happy. God's will for my life is to overflow with happiness. I can have (illness) and still lead a happy life."

Recommended Prayer Time: 10 minutes
Journal: Reflection

Exercise: List ten times you were happy since your diagnosis

Mantra for the day: I am free to be happy.

7. __Compassion__

"I know many people suffer from (illness). I know I am not alone. I know people suffer more than I do in many ways. God please help me to think of others' and not just my own suffering."

Recommended Prayer Time: 15 minutes

Journal: Reflection

Exercise: List some people you know who you would NOT want to trade places with

Mantra for the day: May I have compassion for others.

8. <u>God's Plan</u>

"I trust in God's divine plan for me. This illness is part of my journey. I can still dream big. My creator has great things planned for me."

Recommended Prayer Time: 20 minutes

Journal: Reflection

Exercise: List 5 life goals you have.

Mantra for the day: May I trust in God's divine plan for me.

CHAPTER FOUR

1. <u>Self-identification</u>

"I am not an illness. I am a person living with an illness. Inside me is my true being, perfect and free from illness. I exist above the realm of illness."
Recommended Prayer Time: 5 minutes
Journal: Reflection
Exercise: List 10 things you like about yourself.
Mantra for the day: I am healthy.

You might wonder why the mantra is, "I am healthy." when you are reading a book because you are sick. You must see yourself outside of your illness. You must not self-identify with the illness. Sometimes when someone is diagnosed with an illness, they may have the feeling of being reduced to an invalid. You might think you can accomplish nothing. One may feel that you are reduced to the expression of an illness wreaking havoc on your body, mind, and spirit. As you grow spiritually, you will stop seeing yourself as a person with this illness. Instead you will see yourself as a mother, father, sister, brother, friend, husband, wife, a practitioner of meditation…the list could go on and on. Normally, it could take many years for someone to see themselves as a whole person, not just a disease. However, this program is carefully crafted to introduce you to 8 virtuous meditations constructed to diminish the effects of a disease and it's emotional suffering. It is meant to shift your perspective from one of self-hatred to one of self-love.

You will become grateful for all the other ways in which you are healthy. You can still do many things. Maybe you can walk, see, hear, feel, breathe, exercise, or do many other things. It is possible that for most part, you are free from illness. Maybe you can no longer walk, see, hear, feel or exercise. But you can do many other things. You are somehow reading this book, then you are considering extraordinarily abstract concepts and questions, such as, "How can someone grow spiritually?" Part of your mind or body might be inactive, not working, diseased or removed. However, how is your spirit? Are you poor in spirit or are you rich? How can you change this? Do you want to change this? What is your spiritual landscape like? Repeat the mantra to yourself; "I am healthy."

Remember to be grateful for the measure of health that God has given to you. Remember that in order to change your spiritual landscape you must will it to change. Use the mantra: I am healthy; my spirit is strong; I am resilient. Think positively. We all have things we would want to improve or change in our lives. Don't you think that the man who cannot walk wants to walk? Don't you think that the man who cannot see wants to see? Measure what health you enjoy, what you have, if only it is the breath. Repeat the mantra to yourself: "I am healthy." You will start to see yourself this way and it will change your experience of your own being. Your being will become your well-being. For without spiritual health, how could you enjoy anything else?

2. <u>Gratefulness</u>

"Instead of seeing my illness as a burden, I will be grateful for all that it has brought me. It has brought me many people to support me. It has brought me humility. I can understand other's suffering better. It has brought me back to God."
Recommended Prayer Time: 5 minutes
Journal: Reflection
Exercise: List ten things you are grateful for.
Mantra for the day: I am grateful.

When a diagnosis first comes, it can be hard to see anything but lack. It may feel like there is a lack of health, a lack of love, a lack of sanity, an absence of God. Yet ironically, through living with an illness it is as if God has called you back to him. As you learn to manage your suffering, you begin to slowly see the goodness in things. You may start counting your blessings; and be grateful for a skillful doctor, the joy you feel when you spend time with friends, the support of family or other things. Your perspective, through meditation and prayer, may shift slowly from all bad to a mixed bag - some good and some bad moments. However, through the practice of gratitude meditation you will grow quickly spiritually. As long as you see lack, you will continue to experience lack. If you see abundance, you will experience abundance. This shift in perception is crucial and is the root of so much of what I consider spiritual growth. If you look back on your life, you might find that the times when you had the most fortunate circumstances did not necessarily correspond to the times when you felt most happy or fulfilled. In fact, good circumstances seldom lead to feelings of contentment. In fact, at those times, one may be most concerned with losing what you have. You may even have felt strong feelings of unhappiness. If you were unhappy then, then happiness was a choice. If you could choose now to be happy or unhappy then it is simply that: a choice.

You may begin to experience a sense of humility and union with others (even strangers). Everyone has a story; everyone has negative experiences. No one escapes unscathed. That is to say that no one gets through life without meeting with some form of suffering. It is the nature of life. God challenges us. For you, it came in the form of illness and disease. Next time you see a stranger think, "That person is just like me. They experience suffering. They have a story too. May they grow in

God's grace." Remember to count your blessings, no matter how humble your circumstances. You will paint your grey dreary world with a rainbow of radiant colors that will change your entire experience. After all, where does reality exist? In the outside world, or inside our minds? If you want to change your mood and spirit, don't look to change your circumstances, look to change your experience of those circumstances. Gratitude is the attitude.

3. <u>Love Meditation</u>

"I love my (insert affected body part, or simply "body"). God's light is inside my (insert affected body part, or simply "body"). I can see light healing my (insert affected body part, or simply "body"). My (insert affected body part, or simply "body") is free from disease.

Recommended Prayer Time: 5 minutes
Journal: Reflection
Exercise: List ten things you love about your body.
Mantra for the day: My body is full of light and love.

It is quite easy for life to seem devoid of love when you are suffering from a disease. When someone is first diagnosed, they can be so shell-shocked that they find it difficult to feel the love around them. They only see the blackness of night. You may see your past leading up to the disease and your health as something dead and gone, never to return. You may see your present as one never-ending string of moments to moments that are full of interminable suffering: physical, mental, and emotional. You may see your future as not worthwhile. Your heart may turn to stone and close to any love around you. When you are in pain and suffering, it is important to do meditations on love. You must force your heart to open, force it to blossom once again, and be receptive to the love around you. You must also look for the opportunities to love others. However, initially the most important thing is for you to love yourself and accept yourself despite your illness. For as many wise people say, "How can you love others, if you do not love yourself first?"

When the heart has shriveled and hardened, that is the most important time to open yourself to the fruit of spiritual life, which is love. You can teach the heart to love again. You can show your heart the many ways that you are capable of loving yourself. If you must, ask others why and how they can love you despite your diagnosis. You might find others are able to answer this question much easier than you yourself can. Write these reasons down and post them somewhere you can see them. Record them on a phone and play them for yourself when you feel your heart closed and hardened. Do anything that you can do to grow in your love for yourself. After this, you can search out teachings on lovingkindness; which is a common meditation for Buddhist practitioners. After you love yourself, you can love your family and friends more. Then you may find that one day you feel your heart opening like a late summer rose to the simple visage of a stranger. Your heart will open again just like a rose in full bloom if it lives in the sunlight of love and kindness.

4. <u>Abundance</u>

"I am healthy in many ways. God has blessed my body so that it may function in the way it does now. I can breathe. Therefore, I experience God's creation. I am alive and blessed with abundance."

Recommended Prayer Time: 5 minutes
Journal: Reflection
Exercise: List ten ways in which you are spiritually abundant.
Mantra for the day: I am blessed with abundance.

A spirit of abundance is about wealth in spirit. Cultivate your spirit. Do not concern yourself with worldly circumstances. Of course, this does not mean to neglect them. We must take care of ourselves physically. The physical world has the power to affect us in many ways. However, our spiritual life is the lens through which we experience the physical world. If our soul is a garden with many delicate blooms, how will the physical experience be for us? If our soul is a desert, our physical experience will scorch us to the core. We will burn from the inside out. You may feel like, "How can I not have a desert of a soul? My very life is being torn from me as I lay in this bed!" I sympathize with your situation. You probably feel justified in your anger, in your lack. However, as I wrote before, if you feel lack, your experience will be one of lack. If you feel abundance, you will experience abundance. This is true despite your physical conditions.

You are still breathing. Life is not over. You may feel that your life is like being a prisoner of war. You might feel captive by your disease. If you do not live in a spirit of abundance, then you ARE a prisoner of your illness. You will never be free. Even if you have a terminal diagnosis, don't you want to die a free man or woman? Maybe you have experienced freedom before, as a child or perhaps before disease captured you. You may be tired of living in a prison that was built by your fears and failed expectations. God loves you. He has not abandoned you. Remember the poem, "Footprints"? God is carrying you right now. Let him lead you into the garden of abundance. Live in the sunlight of the spirit. Follow the breath. Cultivate your spirit. Pray. Meditate. Contemplate. Reflect. Be free.

5. <u>Forgiveness</u>

"I forgive myself for having (illness). It is not my fault. I forgive God for making this part of my life. I understand that this is part of my journey to wisdom and freedom."

Recommended Prayer Time: 10 minutes

Journal: Reflection

Exercise: List ten good things that have happened since your diagnosis.

Mantra for the day: Forgiveness leads to

freedom.

When you are first diagnosed, you might have felt like somehow it was your fault. As you grow in your understanding of life, God, and circumstance, you may come to understand that this illness could possibly be a blessing in disguise. When you were healthy, were you obsessed with material goals such as making more money and having a bigger house? Probably the moment you were diagnosed, it changed things completely; it might have made you humble and meek. These were not bad things. Did you have an immediately deeper understanding of other's suffering? Through realizing the good things that have come into your life from the suffering of the illness, allow yourself to forgive yourself for having this disease. It was not your fault. You did not cause this by thinking negative thoughts or having bad karma. It was simply part of God's plan. And please, forgive God for granting you suffering and start to believe that it is all part of God's divine plan for your life.

It may take you years of practice to come to a place of gratitude, abundance, humility, love, forgiveness, compassion, happiness, and an understanding of how this is all part of God's plan. You have started the journey; maybe you have been on this road for a while. This program will provide you the foundation for coming to an understanding of how your illness is just a small part of God's divine plan for you. Forgive yourself, forgive God, and continue your life in a way that leads to freedom and peace. Freedom is God's plan for you today, tomorrow, and for eternity.

6. <u>Happiness</u>

"There are many ways to be happy. There can be suffering in life and I can still be happy. God's will for my life to is overflow with happiness. I can have (illness) and still lead a happy life."
Recommended Prayer Time: 10 minutes
Journal: Reflection
Exercise: List ten times you were happy since your diagnosis.
Mantra for the day: I am free to be happy.

I am free to be happy. What a wonderful thought. There are many ways to be happy. Happiness naturally arises from stillness. Sometimes it seems that happiness is about doing things that bring you joy. While pleasant experiences can bring about feelings of joy or even elation, they only bring intermittent happiness. As you return to your routine, you may experience happiness every time your life returns to normal. However, even then you may still be unhappy. You may be full of fears. Fears that the medicine might stop working, that your illness would return or worsen and that you would be forced into a miserable state by this illness. Therefore, returning to normal does not bring happiness either. Sometimes it only brings with it insurmountable fears. Not until you start on the spiritual path of prayer and meditation will you be able to experience long periods of uninterrupted happiness.

The greatest phenomenon of fruitful spiritual life is when you are happy for no reason at all. You are just experiencing the joy of awakening. In stillness you will find a fountain of joy. Life will cease to be an unending stream of miseries. In time, you might awaken to the mystery of life. Occasionally, you might have negative thoughts or fears about your illness. However, eventually you will be able to dismiss them through the power of a trained mind: a mind focused on the virtues that God has given you to enjoy. The virtues that God has given you to enjoy are what the meditations in this book are based on: happiness, gratefulness, forgiveness, abundance, love, and compassion. Experience these and you will experience everlasting happiness.

7. <u>Compassion</u>

"I know many people suffer from (illness). I know I am not alone. I know people suffer more than I do in many ways. God please help me to think of others' and not just my own suffering."
Recommended Prayer Time: 15 minutes
Journal: Reflection
Exercise: List some people you know who you would NOT want to trade places with
Mantra for the day: May I have compassion for others.

You may think your situation is so bad that you would trade places with anyone else on this green earth. Or you may think that you would trade places with most people. Most people have it better than you. This is a case of the grass is greener on the other side. If you needed to be without illness to be happy and free, then why are some people who are very sick happier than those who are very healthy? Why are some who live in prison happier and freer than some people who live in mansions? Life is a paradox. We are given so much, yet we look at what we don't have. We can't be thin, so we diet. We can't be beautiful, so we have plastic surgery. Forever wanting the thing you cannot have is what you will be doing if you do not recognize the truth in your situation. It is not your illness that plagues you, it is your consistent ignoring of the fruits of the spiritual life. Do not try to think, "Oh, if I just didn't have this illness, my life would be perfect." Realize that these words are not true. You are suffering because of your reaction to your illness, not because of any physical condition.

To practice compassion, try thinking of others. Try to think of how hard their lives are. Think of how difficult it is for them. Cultivate compassion. Your garden will begin to grow. Part of your suffering comes from grasping so hard to your expectations for your health, wealth, house, family, etc. If you only think of yourself, you will fall short with almost every expectation you have. Shift your focus. Think of others. Think of the homeless. Do not think of your fear of being homeless. Think of those who have passed on. Do not fear passing on. Think of those who have suffered more than you. Do not sit around fearing more suffering than you are experiencing. We are all interconnected. We are all playing a part in this human experience. When you tire of your fears and unfulfilled expectations, think of others and their suffering. May I have compassion for others.

8. <u>God's Plan</u>

"I trust in God's divine plan for me. This illness is part of my journey. I can still dream big. My creator has great things planned for me."
Recommended Prayer Time: 20 minutes
Journal: Reflection
Exercise: List 5 life goals you have.
Mantra for the day: May I trust in God's divine plan for me.

Part of recovery or dealing with an illness that is still part of your life is having faith that good things are still in store for you. It is hard to believe when you have so much taken from you, whether it's your physical health, an ability to function at a certain level of productivity or even your sanity, that good things can happen. You only see what you can't do. You see the job you can no longer perform, the college that is now inaccessible to you, the bed you're confined to, the never-ending stream of doctor's appointments and treatments. However, although your life has changed drastically, once you adjust you will find that good things still happen. Babies are still born, people get married, joyful events take place of which you can be a part of.

You must be grateful for the measure of health that God has granted you. You must think of what you do have. From that attitude of gratitude, you will start to see good things in your life occurring also. This book's intention is for you to infuse beautiful, good, and virtuous things into your life. With a dedicated practice you will be able to see the roses among the thorns. I speak from the experience of being torn down, being called back to God and practicing these meditations on virtues. My life improved, but most of it was due to a drastic shift in perspective; from hate to love, from lack to abundance, from resent to gratefulness, from self-pity to seeing myself as a whole person with many blessings. This was God's plan for me, and for you, when he gave you this illness. He is reminding you to see the beauty in life. To live with what you have and find joy in the quiet moments.

Return to prayer, practice meditation, celebrate life, love abundantly, count your blessings, let your heart forgive and you will soon recognize that God has a divine plan for you. He is planning great things for you. He is your ultimate spiritual teacher. Everything he gives is a gift, even if it was the greatest challenge of your life. There is a reason why you are here. There is a reason why he chose this path for you. Now you are the one who must take the first leap of faith. Move out of fear and into faith. Trust in God's divine plan for you. Like many say, "The darkest moment is right before dawn." Step into the sunlight of the spirit. See your illness as part of your journey. It is not a destination. That is not what God intended. Life is still beautiful.

The light in me honors the divine light in you.

Namaste,
Betty Lynn

ABOUT THE AUTHOR

Betty Lynn Tims is an educator, artist, yoga and meditation teacher and writer who resides in a suburb of New York City. She has been practicing yoga for 22 years, but it wasn't until she was diagnosed with a cluster migraine, that she took meditation seriously – devoting 1-2 hours per day to the practice for years. This cleared up her migraines and tension headaches and had many positive effects on her health and well-being. She advocates for mindfulness in the schools and teaches at local yoga studios.

Her blog for book reviews is at inspirationforyourlife.weebly.com. Her artwork portfolio can be found at bettylynntims.com. Her yoga blog can be found at yogaandmeditationbybettylynn.com. Finally, her educational website is mrstimsclass.weebly.com.

Thank you for taking the time to read about her personal journey of healing both physically, mentally, and spiritually. Thank you for dedicating time to becoming a better version of yourself – you are making the world a better place.

Please share this book after reading it with a friend or donate to your local library.